THE HEALING PATH: LESSONS FROM A MENTAL HEALTH PROFESSIONAL

A Practitioner's Insights on Navigating Mental Health and Finding Hope Through Care

McArthur C. C. Okorocha

McARTHUR OKOROCHA has experience in wards, community teams, and is currently pursuing a mental health nursing degree. The purpose of this book is to raise awareness about a variety of mental health conditions you may not be fully aware of, as well as the resources available to help you deal with them. It also contains McArthur's most impactful words and advice, so that you can be empowered to make the change you need, today.

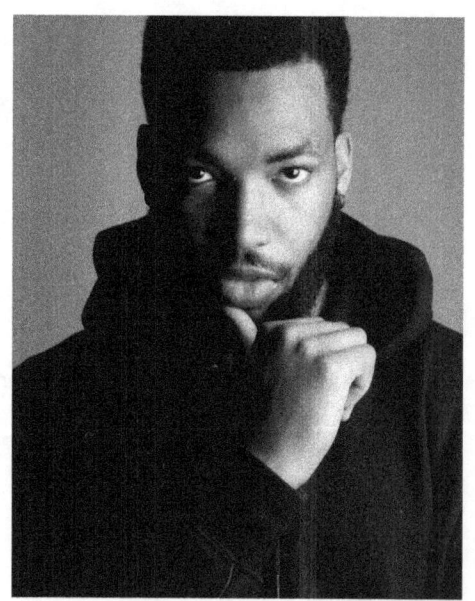

INTRODUCTION

In recent years, the conversation surrounding mental health has grown louder, but for many, the journey toward understanding, healing, and hope remains unclear. As someone who has worked closely with individuals facing various mental health challenges, I have witnessed firsthand the complexities of the human mind and the struggles people face in seeking the support they need.

The Healing Path: Lessons from a Mental Health Professional is the result of years spent on the frontlines of mental health care. In this book, I draw from my experiences as a mental health practitioner, sharing stories, insights, and reflections that I hope will shed light on the diverse mental health challenges people encounter daily. My goal is simple: to help demystify mental health issues and guide readers—whether they are patients, caregivers, or simply individuals looking to understand more—toward finding the support they need.

I have chosen to write this book because I believe that mental health is not just a professional field—it's a personal and human experience we all share. I have worked with individuals from all walks of life, each facing unique battles with their mental well-being, from anxiety and depression to more complex conditions like schizophrenia or bipolar disorder. While no two stories are the same, the common thread that runs through each experience is the need for compassion, understanding, and accessible support.

My hope is that through the chapters of this book, you will find valuable lessons and insights, drawn from both clinical knowledge and personal experience, to help navigate the difficult yet essential conversations about mental health. Whether you are someone living with mental health challenges, a loved one trying to support a person in need, or a professional in the field, I believe there is something here for everyone.

Through this book, I also aim to raise awareness about the broad spectrum of mental health issues that can affect individuals and emphasise the importance of seeking help. Mental health care is not a one-size-fits-all solution. There are a range of therapies, treatments, and support systems available, and I want to show that no matter the struggle, there is a path toward healing.

I invite you to walk this path with me, as we explore the many facets of mental health and the lessons learned along the way. Together, we can contribute to breaking down the stigma and fostering a world where mental health is treated with the same care and respect as physical health. After all, healing begins with understanding, and understanding starts with sharing our stories.

CHAPTER 1: THE SILENT STORM

"Anxiety is like a constant background noise, always there, always intrusive. It's a storm that never passes."

The first time I met Sarah, She was sitting in the corner of her room on the female acute ward, knees tucked to her chest, her breathing shallow and rapid. Her eyes darted nervously, as if searching for an escape from an invisible threat. Her chart indicated a history of extreme anxiety, but seeing her in person made the clinical notes feel distant and inadequate in capturing the depth of her suffering.

Sarah's anxiety was more than just a feeling—it was a visceral, all-encompassing experience that consumed her every moment. She had been admitted to the ward after a severe panic attack that left her immobilised, unable to communicate with her family. Her extreme anxiety had escalated to the point where she could no longer manage daily life.

One evening, a seemingly small incident set off a chain reaction that would test both Sarah and the team's ability to manage her anxiety. The ward had a routine fire alarm test, a standard procedure that we were all used to, but for Sarah, it was a trigger. The sudden loud noise sent her spiralling into a full-blown panic attack.

She ran to the door, desperately pulling at the handle to leave, her breath coming in gasps. She screamed for us to "make it stop" as if the alarm were some kind of torturous weapon. Her hands shook uncontrollably, her body rigid with fear. We immediately rushed to her side, but no amount of comforting words could bring her back to reality at that moment. Her mind was locked in a battle we could not see.

This wasn't just a momentary challenge for Sarah; it was a reflection of the constant internal chaos she experienced. The team and I were faced with the difficult task of grounding her amidst her overwhelming panic, but it took time and patience.

For Sarah, immediate de-escalation was key. We employed a few strategies that had been effective in managing her anxiety in the past:

1. **Grounding Techniques:** First, we focused on bringing her back to the present. Grounding techniques like asking her to focus on her surroundings and identify tangible things—such as the texture of her blanket or the colour of the walls—helped bring her mind back from the brink. We asked her to describe them out loud, giving her mind something to latch onto other than the panic.
2. **Controlled Breathing:** Once Sarah was somewhat responsive, we guided her through deep breathing exercises. Breathing slowly and deliberately, in through the nose and out through the mouth, helped reduce the severity of her hyperventilation. We spoke softly and calmly, matching her breath until she could follow.
3. **Creating a Safe Space:** Sarah's room was her sanctuary on the ward, so we encouraged her to return there once she was more stable. We dimmed the lights and removed any potential distractions, allowing her to calm down in her safe environment.
4. **Medication:** In Sarah's case, she was already prescribed a short-term course of anti-anxiety medication, which

helped ease her symptoms. After this particular incident, we worked closely with the psychiatrist to adjust her treatment plan, ensuring that her medication was carefully monitored and optimised for her needs.

Many of us have felt anxious at some point in our lives—before a big event, an important decision, or a life-changing moment. But imagine feeling that level of anxiety every single day, with no clear cause and no easy solution. For Sarah, this was her reality. Extreme anxiety can make even the most ordinary situations feel overwhelming, like an inescapable storm constantly brewing.

For those struggling with anxiety like Sarah, there is hope, and there are many resources available in the UK to help manage and treat anxiety disorders.

- **NHS Mental Health Services:** The National Health Service (NHS) provides free access to mental health support, including therapy and medication. General practitioners (GPs) are often the first point of contact for those experiencing extreme anxiety, and they can refer patients to specialised mental health services.
- **Cognitive Behavioural Therapy (CBT):** One of the most effective treatments for anxiety is CBT, which helps patients understand and change the patterns of thinking that fuel their anxiety. This therapy is widely available through the NHS and private services.
- **NHS Talking Therapies (formerly IAPT):** For those seeking quicker access to therapy, the **Improving Access to Psychological Therapies (IAPT)** service offers free counselling and therapy sessions aimed at treating anxiety and depression. These services are available in most areas of the UK and can be accessed through a referral from a GP or self-referral.
- **Medication:** In some cases, medication such as **Selective Serotonin Reuptake Inhibitors (SSRIs)** or benzodiazepines may be prescribed to help manage the symptoms of severe

anxiety. It's important for this to be done under careful medical supervision, as was the case with Sarah.
- **Helplines and Support Groups:** For immediate help, helplines like **Anxiety UK** or **Mind** offer telephone and online support for individuals struggling with anxiety. Support groups, both in-person and online, provide a space for people to share their experiences and coping strategies with others who understand their challenges.

* * *

In this chapter, we've explored Sarah's experience with extreme anxiety—an experience that, for many, can feel debilitating. But it's important to remember that anxiety is manageable, and there are a variety of resources and strategies available to help people regain control of their lives. Whether through therapy, medication, or support systems, no one has to face anxiety alone.

* * *

In the next chapter, we'll dive into another mental health challenge—one that is often misunderstood and stigmatised: bipolar. Just as with anxiety, there are many faces to bipolar, and understanding its nuances is key to providing the right support.

CHAPTER 2: THE PENDULUM OF THE MIND

"Bipolar disorder is like living on a seesaw, constantly swinging between extremes. The challenge is learning how to stay balanced when the ground is always shifting."

I once worked with a service user named "Mark". He was pacing the corridor of the ward, his eyes wide with excitement, talking rapidly about a new business idea that he was certain would "change the world." His energy was infectious, but there was something unsettling about the intensity with which he spoke. Mark had been diagnosed with Bipolar Disorder, and he was in the midst of a manic episode. While his mind was racing at an extraordinary pace, the reality around him was starting to blur.

Not long after Mark's admission, we encountered a significant challenge. One morning, Mark woke up unusually early and immediately began making demands—he wanted access to his phone, a laptop, and a whiteboard to map out his business ideas. When the ward rules about restricted use of electronics were explained to him, Mark became increasingly agitated. His frustration quickly escalated into anger. He stormed into the communal area, knocking over chairs and shouting at the staff, convinced that we were sabotaging his success.

For the team, it was a delicate situation. We had to balance his safety, the safety of the other patients, and Mark's heightened state of mania. The energy in the room was tense, and we knew that one wrong move could escalate the situation even further.

Managing Mark's episode required a multifaceted approach, as dealing with the highs of mania can be just as challenging as managing the lows of depression.

1. **Calm Communication:** The first step was calming Mark through communication. We spoke to him in a low, steady tone, avoiding confrontation or engaging with the grandiose ideas that were fueling his mania. Instead, we focused on grounding him, reminding him of where he was and the importance of following the ward's structure.
2. **Time and Space:** To de-escalate the situation, we encouraged Mark to spend time in his room, which was quieter and less stimulating. The acute ward can often feel overwhelming during a manic episode, so creating a controlled environment helped ease his agitation.
3. **Medication Management:** Bipolar disorder often requires a combination of mood stabilisers and antipsychotics to manage both manic and depressive episodes. After consulting with the psychiatrist, Mark's medication was adjusted to better control his manic symptoms. The team monitored his reaction closely, making sure the side effects were manageable and that his mood gradually stabilised.
4. **Structured Routine:** Mark's mania thrived on chaos, so we introduced more structure into his day. Regular meals, scheduled therapeutic activities, and daily check-ins with the staff helped him feel more anchored. This structure played a crucial role in bringing him back from the manic high he was experiencing.

Bipolar disorder is a condition that many misunderstand. The extremes of mania and depression can feel like two entirely different worlds, and for those living with the condition, the rapid swings between these emotional states can be exhausting. Mania, in particular, can make someone feel invincible—until the inevitable crash comes. For Mark, it wasn't just a matter of managing his highs and lows but finding a way to live in the middle, where stability felt foreign.

For those who, like Mark, live with Bipolar Disorder, there are several resources and treatments available in the UK to help manage the condition effectively.

- **NHS Mental Health Services:** The NHS offers comprehensive support for individuals diagnosed with Bipolar Disorder. Treatment typically involves a combination of medication, psychotherapy, and regular monitoring through community mental health teams (CMHTs).
- **Mood Stabilizers and Antipsychotics:** Medication is often essential in managing the extreme mood swings associated with Bipolar Disorder. **Lithium** is one of the most commonly prescribed mood stabilisers, along with **antipsychotic medications** like olanzapine or quetiapine to control mania. The NHS provides access to these medications, which are regularly reviewed to ensure efficacy.
- **Psychotherapy:** Cognitive Behavioural Therapy (CBT) can help individuals with Bipolar Disorder recognize the patterns of their illness and develop strategies to manage both the depressive and manic phases. The NHS offers access to CBT through primary care services or referral from a GP.
- **Crisis Teams:** For those experiencing severe mood episodes, NHS **Crisis Teams** provide immediate support in the community to prevent hospital admissions where possible. These teams can intervene during manic or depressive episodes, providing urgent care and guidance.
- **Support Networks and Charities:** Organisations like **Bipolar UK** offer valuable resources, including peer support

groups, educational materials, and a helpline. These services can be critical for individuals and families navigating life with Bipolar Disorder, offering a sense of community and understanding.

❋ ❋ ❋

In this chapter, we've delved into Mark's experience with Bipolar Disorder, specifically focusing on the challenges of managing mania in a ward setting. While Bipolar Disorder can be difficult to manage, the right combination of medication, structured routines, and therapy can bring stability and allow individuals to lead fulfilling lives.

❋ ❋ ❋

In the next chapter, we'll shift focus to a different aspect of mental health—schizophrenia, a condition that is often shrouded in stigma and misunderstanding. Through the story of another patient, we'll explore the realities of living with this complex condition and the paths available toward recovery.

CHAPTER 3: BEHIND THE VEIL

> *"Schizophrenia is not just hearing voices—it's living in a reality that feels disconnected from the world others know. It's a constant battle to distinguish what is real from what is imagined."*

This chapter focuses on James. Upon my first contact with James, he was sitting at the edge of his bed, his gaze fixed on something that wasn't there. He occasionally mumbled under his breath, seemingly in conversation with an unseen entity. James had been living with schizophrenia for years, cycling in and out of psychiatric care, often brought back to the acute ward when his symptoms became unmanageable.

Schizophrenia had stolen much of his sense of security and trust in the world around him. The lines between reality and delusion were blurred for James, and his paranoia, hallucinations, and disorganised thinking made it difficult for him to feel safe, even in the structured environment of the ward.

One morning, James came to the nurse's station, visibly agitated. He claimed that people in the ward were plotting against him and that the television was sending him coded messages about a plan to harm him. His paranoia was escalating quickly, and his behaviour was becoming unpredictable. He refused to return to his room, insisting that the only way to "protect himself" was to stay near the exit door.

The challenge for our team was managing his growing distress without further inflaming his delusions. Schizophrenia is a condition that can be deeply isolating, especially when someone believes that the world is conspiring against them. Our priority was to ensure his safety and help him regain a sense of calm, but this required sensitivity and careful communication.

Managing James' schizophrenia required a combination of immediate de-escalation and long-term therapeutic strategies. Each step was crucial in helping him manage his symptoms and reconnect with reality.

1. **Non-Confrontational Communication:** We knew that confronting James' delusions directly could increase his paranoia, so we focused on validating his feelings without reinforcing his fears. Instead of arguing with him about the television messages or the perceived plot against him, we reassured him that he was safe and that we were there to support him.
2. **Quiet Environment:** Schizophrenia, especially when accompanied by paranoia and auditory hallucinations, can be exacerbated by overstimulation. We guided James to a quieter area of the ward, away from the common room and the television, to reduce the external stimuli that were fueling his distress.
3. **Medication Management:** Schizophrenia often requires antipsychotic medication to manage symptoms. James had been prescribed medication, but during his stay, the psychiatrist adjusted his dosage to better target his delusions and hallucinations. This adjustment took time, as finding the right balance of medication is essential for stabilising patients without causing too many side effects.
4. **Building Trust:** One of the most critical components of James' care was building a relationship based on trust. Schizophrenia often leaves individuals feeling

isolated and misunderstood, so consistent, empathetic communication was vital. Over time, we developed a rapport with James, and he began to rely on the team for reassurance when his delusions became overwhelming.

For many of us, reality is something we take for granted—it's stable, predictable, and shared by those around us. But for individuals like James, schizophrenia distorts that reality, making even the simplest interactions feel fraught with danger or deceit. It's not just about hearing voices or seeing things that aren't there; it's about living in a world where trust is elusive, and every moment is overshadowed by fear or confusion.

Schizophrenia is a lifelong condition, but with the right support, individuals can lead stable and fulfilling lives. In the UK, several resources are available to help manage the symptoms of schizophrenia and provide long-term care.

- **NHS Mental Health Services:** The NHS offers comprehensive treatment for schizophrenia, including medication, therapy, and community-based support. Patients typically work with a **Community Mental Health Team (CMHT)** to receive ongoing care and monitoring.
- **Antipsychotic Medications:** Medications such as **olanzapine**, **risperidone**, or **clozapine** are commonly used to manage the symptoms of schizophrenia. These medications help reduce delusions, hallucinations, and disorganised thinking, though they must be carefully monitored for side effects.
- **Cognitive Behavioral Therapy for Psychosis (CBTp):** CBTp is a specialised form of therapy available through the NHS that helps individuals with schizophrenia challenge and manage their delusions and hallucinations. It's particularly effective when combined with medication.
- **Early Intervention Services:** For those in the early stages of schizophrenia, **Early Intervention in Psychosis (EIP)** teams provide targeted support to help individuals manage their

symptoms and prevent long-term disability. These services are critical in reducing the impact of the illness and promoting recovery.

- **Support Networks and Charities:** Charities like **Rethink Mental Illness** and **SANE** provide educational resources, support groups, and helplines for individuals living with schizophrenia and their families. These organisations offer practical advice and a sense of community for those affected by the disorder.

※ ※ ※

In this chapter, we've explored James' experience with schizophrenia—a condition that can feel like living in a constant state of uncertainty and fear. While schizophrenia can be a challenging disorder to manage, there are effective treatments and support systems available in the UK that can help individuals like James lead stable and meaningful lives.

※ ※ ※

In the next chapter, we will explore another complex mental health issue: Depression. Through the story of another patient, we'll discuss the challenges and misconceptions surrounding these disorders and the available treatments.

CHAPTER 4: THE WEIGHT OF THE WORLD

"Depression is not just sadness; it's a deep, unshakable heaviness that can make even the smallest of tasks feel impossible. It's not simply feeling down—it's feeling like the world has lost all colour."

The story of David is quite an interesting one. His presence on the ward was almost ghost-like. He sat slumped in his chair, eyes vacant, his voice barely above a whisper. There was a profound stillness to him, as if he had withdrawn so far into himself that even his surroundings felt distant. David had been admitted to the ward after an unsuccessful suicide attempt, and his depression was so severe that he could barely muster the energy to eat, let alone engage in conversation.

Depression is a silent, suffocating illness that often hides behind a mask of normalcy. But for David, it had stripped away everything—his motivation, his joy, and even his will to keep going. He had been living in this darkness for so long that the idea of getting better seemed like a cruel joke.

One afternoon, the team noticed that David hadn't left his room all day. This wasn't entirely unusual, given his deep depression, but there was something about his absence that felt unsettling.

When I went to check on him, I found David sitting on the edge of his bed, staring at a bottle of painkillers he had hidden in his jacket. He wasn't actively taking them, but the intent was clear—he had been contemplating ending his life again.

At that moment, time seemed to stand still. The challenge wasn't just keeping David physically safe—it was finding a way to reach him emotionally, to show him that there was still hope, even though he couldn't see it. He was trapped in his own mind, and no amount of reasoning could pull him out of the dark hole he had fallen into.

The team quickly intervened, but the emotional gravity of that moment weighed heavily on all of us. David's pain was palpable, and it was clear that he wasn't just battling depression—he was battling the overwhelming desire to escape from a world that felt unbearable.

Helping David wasn't just about responding to this particular incident. It was about providing ongoing support to help him slowly emerge from the fog of depression. The following steps were crucial in his care:

1. **Immediate Safety Measures:** After the incident, we took immediate steps to ensure David's safety, including removing any potential means of harm and increasing his observation level. This wasn't about taking away his autonomy, but rather about protecting him during this vulnerable time.
2. **One-on-One Engagement:** Depression can isolate patients from the world around them, making even the simplest human interactions feel exhausting. I started spending time with David one-on-one, not pressuring him to talk, but simply sitting with him, offering a quiet presence. Over time, he began to open up, sharing small snippets of his life—his love for music, the career he had lost, the relationships that had fractured under the weight of his illness.

3. **Antidepressant Medication:** Like many people suffering from severe depression, David was prescribed antidepressants. In his case, **Selective Serotonin Reuptake Inhibitors (SSRIs)** were introduced to help regulate his mood. This was done carefully, as the early stages of antidepressant treatment can sometimes increase suicidal thoughts before the medication begins to have a positive effect.
4. **Therapeutic Interventions:** In addition to medication, we worked with David to start **Cognitive Behavioural Therapy (CBT)** sessions. CBT focuses on identifying and challenging the negative thought patterns that fuel depression. In David's case, it was crucial to help him break free from the belief that nothing could change for the better.
5. **Structured Routine:** One of the most effective strategies for managing depression is creating structure in a patient's day. David was encouraged to participate in small, achievable tasks, such as attending group therapy or going for a short walk in the hospital garden. These activities, while seemingly insignificant, played a critical role in helping him rebuild a sense of normalcy and routine.

We've all had days where getting out of bed feels like an impossible task, where the weight of life's challenges presses down on us. But for those like David, depression isn't just a bad day—it's an unrelenting, all-encompassing state of despair that can last for weeks, months, or even years. The hardest part is often that depression lies to you. It tells you that nothing will ever get better, that you're alone, and that the world would be better off without you. But that's not the truth, even though it feels like it.

Depression is one of the most common mental health issues in the UK, but it's also one of the most treatable. Whether through therapy, medication, or a combination of approaches, there is help available for those who need it.

- **NHS Mental Health Services:** The NHS offers free access to mental health support, including therapy and medication for individuals suffering from depression. **GPs** are often the first point of contact and can refer patients to specialised mental health services when needed.
- **Medication:** Antidepressants like **SSRIs (Selective Serotonin Reuptake Inhibitors)** are commonly prescribed to help balance brain chemistry and alleviate the symptoms of depression. For more severe cases, **SNRIs (Serotonin-Norepinephrine Reuptake Inhibitors)** or other medications might be used. These are available through the NHS, and treatment is closely monitored to ensure effectiveness.
- **Talking Therapies:** NHS Talking Therapies (formerly IAPT) provide free counselling and therapy services, including **Cognitive Behavioural Therapy (CBT)**, which is one of the most effective treatments for depression. These services are accessible via self-referral or a GP referral.
- **Crisis Support:** For individuals experiencing a mental health crisis, **NHS Crisis Teams** are available to provide immediate support in the community. These teams can intervene during a severe depressive episode and offer urgent care to prevent hospital admission.
- **Helplines and Support Groups:** Charities like **Samaritans, Mind,** and **CALM (Campaign Against Living Miserably)** offer 24/7 helplines for individuals struggling with depression and suicidal thoughts. These services provide a lifeline for those in immediate need of support, offering someone to talk to when the darkness feels overwhelming.

* * *

In this chapter, we've explored David's battle with depression—a battle that left him feeling hopeless and unable to see a future for himself. Depression is an illness that distorts reality, making it hard to believe that things can get better. But with the right support, treatment, and time, recovery is possible.

❊ ❊ ❊

In the next chapter, we'll explore another mental health issue that often goes unnoticed: post-traumatic stress disorder (PTSD). Through the story of a patient who struggled with this condition, we'll delve into the long-lasting effects of trauma and the journey toward healing.

CHAPTER 5: SHADOWS OF THE PAST

"Trauma leaves a mark, not just on the body but on the mind. For those who've faced the unimaginable, the battle doesn't end when the danger is over—it continues, replaying over and over in the mind like an unrelenting film."

Jennifer was a military veteran who had faced the horrors of war head-on. On the surface, she seemed calm and composed—just another person going about her day. But beneath that exterior was a woman haunted by memories too painful to escape. Jennifer had been discharged from service after witnessing a traumatic event that she could never forget, and although her body had survived the war, her mind had not. She was living with **Post-Traumatic Stress Disorder (PTSD)**, and every day was a battle against the flashbacks, nightmares, and overwhelming anxiety that dominated her life.

I met Jennifer whilst I was on placement with the community mental health team, where we worked to support individuals with severe mental health conditions outside of the hospital setting. Jennifer's case was one that particularly resonated with me because it showed just how profoundly trauma can impact a person long after the event is over. Her war might have ended, but in her mind, it was still raging.

One afternoon, during a routine home visit, we arrived at Jennifer's house to find her in the grip of a full-blown flashback.

She was crouched in the corner of her living room, her breathing rapid, her eyes wide with fear. To her, she wasn't in the safety of her home anymore—she was back on the battlefield, surrounded by the chaos and violence of war. She kept repeating, "They're coming, they're coming," her voice trembling with terror.

This was one of the most challenging moments I experienced on placement. It wasn't just about calming Jennifer down—it was about bringing her back to the present, to a reality that felt far away from where her mind had taken her. The team knew that we couldn't force her out of the flashback, but instead, we needed to gently guide her back, step by step.

Working with Jennifer and supporting her through these moments required a comprehensive and sensitive approach, particularly because we were caring for her in the community, outside of the controlled environment of a hospital.

1. **Grounding Techniques:** During the flashback, our immediate goal was to help Jennifer reconnect with the present. We used grounding techniques—simple, sensory-focused exercises designed to pull her out of the traumatic memory. We asked her to focus on the textures around her, like the fabric of the couch she was sitting on, and the sounds in the room, like the ticking of the clock, to remind her where she was. These small details helped her distinguish the here and now from the memories of the battlefield.
2. **Building Trust:** PTSD often shatters trust, particularly for those who have experienced trauma in high-stakes environments like the military. Building a relationship with Jennifer based on consistency, patience, and understanding was essential. She needed to feel safe enough to share her experiences with us, and that trust was something we nurtured over time through our visits and check-ins.
3. **Trauma-Focused Therapy:** Jennifer was undergoing

Trauma-Focused Cognitive Behavioural Therapy (TF-CBT), one of the most effective treatments for PTSD. As part of our role in the community team, we supported her therapy journey by reinforcing the coping strategies she was learning. This included helping her practise relaxation techniques and positive self-talk during our sessions.

4. **Medication Management:** Like many PTSD patients, Jennifer was prescribed **Selective Serotonin Reuptake Inhibitors (SSRIs)** to help manage her symptoms of anxiety and depression. Additionally, **Prazosin** was prescribed to reduce her nightmares, which were a significant part of her PTSD. As part of her care, we monitored her progress with these medications, ensuring that they were effective without causing too many side effects.

5. **Social Support and Routine:** Jennifer had become isolated since her return from the military, withdrawing from friends and family out of fear that they wouldn't understand her experiences. One of our goals in the community team was to help her rebuild those connections and encourage her to engage with veteran support groups. Gradually, Jennifer began to attend weekly meetings with other veterans, which became an important part of her recovery.

For many people, trauma is an abstract concept, something that happens to others. But for those like Jennifer, trauma is a constant companion, dictating her thoughts, emotions, and actions. PTSD doesn't just bring back memories—it makes the past feel immediate, as if the danger never left. For veterans and others who've experienced severe trauma, it's not just about surviving the event, but learning how to live with the aftermath.

In the UK, PTSD is a recognised and treatable condition, but it requires the right combination of therapy, medication, and support to manage effectively. The following resources are available to individuals suffering from PTSD:

- **NHS Mental Health Services:** PTSD treatment is available through the NHS, with specialised **Trauma-Focused Cognitive Behavioural Therapy (TF-CBT)** being the gold standard for care. **Eye Movement Desensitization and Reprocessing (EMDR)** is another therapy that is commonly offered to help individuals process traumatic memories.
- **Medication:** SSRIs are often prescribed to help with the depression and anxiety associated with PTSD, while **Prazosin** can be used to reduce nightmares. These medications are available through the NHS, and patients can access them with the guidance of their GP or psychiatrist.
- **Veteran-Specific Services:** For individuals like Jennifer who are military veterans, specialised support services are available. **Combat Stress** is a leading UK charity that provides mental health support to veterans, offering therapy, rehabilitation, and community programs specifically designed for those who have served in the military. Additionally, the **Veterans' Mental Health Transition, Intervention and Liaison Service (TILS)** provides NHS mental health services tailored to veterans and their families.
- **Support Groups and Charities:** Charities like **Mind** and **Rethink Mental Illness** offer peer support groups and helplines, where individuals can connect with others who have experienced trauma. For veterans, there are also specific groups like **Help for Heroes**, which provide social, financial, and mental health support for those who have served.

* * *

In this chapter, we've explored Jennifer's struggle with PTSD, a condition that left her trapped between her past and present. For individuals like Jennifer, trauma doesn't fade with time—it lingers, impacting every facet of daily life. But with the right care, support, and strategies, it's possible to begin the journey toward healing.

❊ ❊ ❊

In the next chapter, we'll turn our attention to a different, but equally complex, mental health challenge: addiction. Through the story of another patient, we'll explore how mental health and substance abuse are often intertwined, and the resources available to break the cycle of addiction.

CHAPTER 6: BENEATH THE SURFACE

> *"Addiction is often hidden beneath layers of shame, denial, and guilt. It's not just a personal struggle—it affects families, communities, and relationships. But for those who fall into its grasp, the path to recovery is often long and filled with obstacles."*

Ama—- I was struck by her gentle demeanour and the weight of her story. As the wife of a well-respected pastor in the Ghanaian community, she carried an image of poise and grace. To the outside world, she was a beacon of strength, a pillar in her church, and a figure of support for her congregation. But behind closed doors, Ama was fighting a hidden battle—an addiction to alcohol that had taken control of her life.

Ama's struggle with addiction was compounded by the cultural and societal expectations placed on her. As a pastor's wife, she felt immense pressure to uphold a standard of perfection, never allowing herself to show weakness or vulnerability. The stress of this role, combined with personal trauma, led her to turn to alcohol as a way of numbing the emotional pain. Over time, what had started as an occasional escape became a dependency that she couldn't shake, and it was destroying her from the inside out.

One evening, during a routine follow-up visit, I arrived at Ama's home to find her in a state of distress. Her hands trembled as she tried to steady herself, the scent of alcohol lingering in the air despite her attempts to hide it. That day, her husband had discovered empty bottles hidden in their house, and the confrontation had left her emotionally shattered. She spoke in hushed tones, her voice breaking with shame as she admitted, "I don't know how to stop. I've prayed, I've begged God, but I can't stop."

This was one of the most challenging moments for me as part of the community team. The tension in her household was palpable, and the stakes were high. Ama's addiction wasn't just affecting her—it was eroding the very foundation of her marriage, her role in the church, and her standing in the community. Yet, she felt trapped, unable to reach out for help in fear of judgement from those closest to her.

The challenge here wasn't just about addressing the physical aspects of Ama's addiction. It was about confronting the deep-rooted emotional and cultural stigmas that made her feel like she had to suffer in silence.

Supporting Ama required a holistic approach, one that took into account not just her physical dependency on alcohol but the emotional, spiritual, and cultural factors contributing to her addiction.

1. **Creating a Safe Space:** The first step in Ama's recovery was providing her with a safe, non-judgmental space where she could be honest about her struggles. Given her position in the community and her fear of being judged, this was crucial. As a team, we reassured her that seeking help was not a sign of failure, but a brave step toward healing. By building trust with Ama, we gave her the courage to open up, something she had been unable to do with her family and church.
2. **Detox and Physical Care:** Ama's addiction had reached a point where detox was necessary to manage the withdrawal symptoms. We worked with her to arrange for a medically supervised detox program. This involved

coordinating with her GP and the local substance misuse services to ensure that she received the proper care during the process, minimising the physical risks associated with alcohol withdrawal.

3. **Culturally Sensitive Therapy:** One of the most important aspects of Ama's care was addressing the cultural stigma surrounding addiction in her community. We referred her to a counsellor who specialised in culturally sensitive care, someone who understood the unique pressures she faced as a Ghanaian woman and a pastor's wife. Through **Cognitive Behavioural Therapy (CBT)**, Ama began to unravel the underlying emotional pain that had fueled her addiction, while also learning healthier coping mechanisms.

4. **Spiritual Support:** Ama's faith was central to her identity, and it was important that her recovery included this aspect of her life. We encouraged her to seek spiritual counselling alongside her therapy, integrating her faith into her healing process. This was not about using religion as a crutch but about allowing her to reconcile her spirituality with her addiction. With the support of a trusted, non-judgmental church member, Ama was able to slowly open up within her faith community, finding a balance between her personal recovery and her role as a pastor's wife.

5. **Family Involvement and Education:** Addiction doesn't just affect the individual—it impacts the entire family. Ama's husband had been left in shock by her admission, struggling to understand how the woman he knew could be battling such a demon. We arranged family therapy sessions, where both Ama and her husband could begin to heal the rifts in their relationship, addressing the secrecy and mistrust that had built up over time. It was crucial for her husband to understand that addiction is an illness, not a moral failing, and that

recovery is a journey that requires support, not shame.

Addiction doesn't discriminate—it affects people from all walks of life, including those we'd least expect. Ama's story highlights how cultural and societal pressures can drive individuals to suffer in silence, hiding their pain behind closed doors. For those in similar situations, it's important to remember that addiction isn't a personal failing, but a condition that requires support, understanding, and treatment.

Addiction is a significant public health issue, but in the UK, there are numerous resources available to help individuals recover and rebuild their lives.

- **NHS Substance Misuse Services:** The NHS provides a range of services for individuals struggling with alcohol and drug addiction, including detox programs, counselling, and rehabilitation services. These are available through GP referrals or self-referral to local substance misuse teams.
- **Alcoholics Anonymous (AA): AA** is a well-known support group that offers free, peer-led meetings for individuals dealing with alcohol addiction. The **12-step program** provides a structured approach to recovery, focusing on community support and personal accountability.
- **Culturally Sensitive Support:** For individuals like Ama, who come from cultural backgrounds where addiction carries significant stigma, organisations like **BAME in Recovery** offer tailored support, focusing on culturally relevant care and understanding the unique challenges faced by ethnic minority communities.
- **Residential Rehab Programs:** For those with severe addictions, residential rehabilitation programs provide an intensive, immersive environment for recovery. These programs offer medical detox, therapy, and life skills training to help individuals rebuild their lives away from the triggers of addiction.
- **Family Support:** Organisations like **Al-Anon** provide

support for families affected by addiction, offering a safe space for loved ones to share their experiences and learn how to support their family member's recovery without enabling destructive behaviours.

※ ※ ※

In this chapter, we've explored Ama's battle with addiction—a battle complicated by her role in her community and the cultural stigmas she faced. Her story is a reminder that addiction doesn't always fit the stereotypes we see in the media. It can touch the lives of people who seem to have it all together, but who are quietly suffering behind closed doors.

※ ※ ※

In the next chapter, we'll dive into the complexities of eating disorders, following the story of another patient who struggled with their relationship with food. Eating disorders are often misunderstood and dismissed, but they are serious mental health conditions that require specialised care.

CHAPTER 7: TWISTED REFLECTIONS

"Eating disorders are often silent, hidden beneath layers of shame, control, and confusion. For many, it starts as a desire for control, but quickly spirals into an overwhelming force that consumes every part of life. It's not just about food—it's about pain, identity, and self-worth."

I met Hannah and Sophie, identical twins who arrived at the **CAMHS (Child and Adolescent Mental Health Services)** ward, suffering from severe eating disorders. On the surface, they appeared almost indistinguishable—same features, same body language, same soft-spoken voices. But behind those identical faces were two separate battles. The twins had been caught in the grip of **Anorexia Nervosa** for years, their lives shrinking around them as they spiralled deeper into the disorder.

The most striking thing about their story was the way their eating disorders mirrored each other, yet diverged in subtle but profound ways. It wasn't uncommon for twins to share similar experiences, especially when it came to mental health, but for Hannah and Sophie, their bond was inseparable in both their suffering and their recovery.

Hannah, the more outgoing of the two, had been the first to show signs of an eating disorder, her weight dropping rapidly after starting secondary school. Sophie, initially unaffected, began to follow her sister's behaviours out of fear and confusion.

Soon, their shared struggle became their reality. Both girls were becoming experts in hiding their condition, crafting a facade of normalcy to those around them, while secretly slipping deeper into isolation and self-doubt.

I'll never forget one particular morning on the CAMHS ward. It was breakfast time, and the twins sat at opposite ends of the dining table, barely speaking. Hannah picked at her food, using her fork to move her scrambled eggs around, while Sophie sat stiffly, her plate untouched. It was clear they were in a deep internal battle, one that they couldn't escape, not even in the safety of the hospital.

Then, without warning, Sophie began to shake violently. She clutched her stomach, tears streaming down her face. The nurses quickly gathered around her, and we immediately rushed her to her room. She was having what seemed like an emotional breakdown, triggered by the prospect of eating. This was the nature of eating disorders—they affected not just the body but the mind, creating an overwhelming fear of food and weight gain. Watching the two sisters struggle simultaneously, each trapped in their own version of fear, was heartbreaking.

The challenge wasn't just in helping Sophie through the moment—it was in understanding how intertwined their recovery was. If one twin fell behind, the other followed. Their journey would need to be handled with extraordinary sensitivity, taking into account both their shared experience and their individual needs.

Working with Hannah and Sophie required a delicate balance. Their eating disorders weren't just about food; they were about control, perfectionism, and an intense desire to meet certain expectations. The following approaches were central to their recovery:

1. **Individualised Therapy with a Shared Focus:** Although the twins' disorders mirrored each other, their paths to recovery needed to be individual. We arranged for

both of them to attend **Cognitive Behavioural Therapy (CBT)**, tailored for eating disorders. CBT helps to challenge the distorted thoughts that often fuel eating disorders, such as the belief that being thin is the only way to be acceptable or that food is the enemy. While their sessions were separate, we made sure to occasionally hold joint sessions so that they could communicate openly about their struggles without feeling pressured by their sister's progress.

2. **Family Therapy:** One of the most important components of their treatment was involving their family in the process. Hannah and Sophie's parents were understandably distressed, confused, and struggling to support their daughters. **Family-Based Therapy (FBT)**, also known as the **Maudsley Method**, was introduced to help the family understand the disorder and become active participants in their children's recovery. Involving the parents wasn't about blaming them—it was about creating an environment where the girls could feel understood and supported. Their family was also educated on how to model healthy eating behaviours, as well as how to handle meal times without confrontation.

3. **Nutritional Therapy and Weight Restoration:** It was crucial that both girls received expert nutritional advice to help restore their physical health. Under the guidance of a dietitian, they were put on a carefully controlled meal plan designed to restore their weight slowly, allowing their bodies to heal from the malnutrition caused by their eating disorders. Meal times were monitored closely, and it was important to support them emotionally through the process. This wasn't just about eating—it was about reconnecting with their bodies and learning to trust that food could nourish them rather than harm them.

4. **Developing Healthy Coping Mechanisms:** Eating

disorders often serve as a coping mechanism for deeper emotional pain or distress. For Hannah and Sophie, learning to cope with stress, anxiety, and their feelings of inadequacy was key to their recovery. They were taught mindfulness techniques, grounding exercises, and ways to reframe negative thoughts. Additionally, we introduced them to **art therapy**, where they were able to express their emotions through creativity, bypassing the difficulty of verbalising their feelings.

5. **Social Support and Group Therapy:** One of the most important aspects of recovery for both girls was finding a sense of belonging outside of the confines of their family and the hospital. We introduced them to support groups for young people with eating disorders, where they could meet others who shared similar struggles. These groups provided a space for them to express their fears and successes without judgement and were instrumental in helping them feel less isolated.

For many young people struggling with eating disorders, there is a desire to be in control—control over food, body image, and how they present themselves to the world. For Hannah and Sophie, their shared struggle meant that they could understand each other's pain, but it also made recovery harder. Eating disorders often affect not just the person but also those around them. For parents, teachers, and friends, it's important to understand that helping someone recover from an eating disorder isn't just about encouraging them to eat—it's about supporting their emotional, psychological, and physical healing.

Eating disorders are complex mental health conditions that require specialised care. In the UK, there are a variety of resources available for those affected by disorders like anorexia, bulimia, and binge eating:

- **NHS Specialist Eating Disorder Units:** The NHS provides specialist treatment for eating disorders through

both inpatient and outpatient units. The treatment usually includes a combination of psychological therapies like **Cognitive Behavioural Therapy (CBT)** and **Family-Based Therapy (FBT)**, as well as medical and nutritional support.
- **Beat - Eating Disorder Charity: Beat** is the UK's leading eating disorder charity, offering support and information for those suffering from eating disorders. They provide helplines, online chat services, and support groups for both individuals and their families. Beat also runs a network of **online recovery communities**, where people can share their experiences and support one another.
- **Community Mental Health Services (CAMHS):** For young people like Hannah and Sophie, **CAMHS** is a valuable resource. CAMHS provides mental health support to children and adolescents who are dealing with a range of mental health challenges, including eating disorders. They offer specialised care, including therapy and support groups tailored for young people.
- **Residential Treatment Programs:** For severe cases, there are a number of **residential treatment programs** available in the UK, where young people can stay for an extended period to receive intensive therapy and support. These programs offer a structured, safe environment for recovery.
- **The National Centre for Eating Disorders:** This private organisation offers a range of treatments, including **CBT** and **interpersonal therapy** (IPT), for both children and adults suffering from eating disorders.

※ ※ ※

In this chapter, we've explored the deeply intertwined experience of twins struggling with eating disorders. Their journey was one of both shared pain and individual resilience. Eating disorders are rarely about food—they are about emotional pain, self-identity, and control. But with the right support, recovery is possible.

※ ※ ※

In the next chapter, we'll turn to a different mental health struggle —one that involves the balance of mind and body: **chronic pain and its psychological effects**. For many individuals, pain is not just a physical experience, but a mental one, affecting every aspect of their lives.

CHAPTER 8: THE UNSEEN BATTLE

> *"Chronic pain is a relentless companion that shadows you, draining your energy, robbing your joy, and quietly whispering that you are no longer in control. But what's often forgotten is that this pain doesn't just affect the body—it invades the mind as well."*

Mr. Turner — He was sitting by the window in the day room of the elderly ward, looking out at the garden with an almost distant expression. He was a tall man, well into his late seventies, his skin thin from years of life and medical treatment. Despite his frail appearance, his presence felt strong—yet his eyes revealed the deep pain that seemed to define his days.

Turner had spent years living with chronic pain following a series of failed surgeries after an accident in his younger years. His lower back and hips were constantly in agony, leaving him barely able to move without assistance. The physical limitations were bad enough, but what was more concerning was the way his pain had slowly taken a psychological toll. His mood had become increasingly withdrawn, his demeanour bleak. He had started to show signs of **depression**, feeling like a burden to his family, his life reduced to a series of pain management appointments and hospital visits.

One particular morning, I was walking through the ward when I heard raised voices coming from Turner's room. I quickly approached to find him shouting at the nursing assistant who was trying to help him into his chair. His pain was flaring up, and his frustration had boiled over. He was refusing to take his medication, angry at the world, angry at his body, and most of all, angry at himself.

"I can't live like this anymore!" he exclaimed, his voice trembling with both anger and sadness. "I'm just a burden to everyone! They don't know what it's like... to live like this, every single day!"

The scene was painful to witness. As his pain intensified, so did his feelings of helplessness and isolation. For Mr. Turner, his pain wasn't just physical—it was psychological. It made him feel worthless, like he was no longer able to live a life worth living. This was a powerful reminder that chronic pain in the elderly doesn't just affect the body; it deeply affects one's mental state, leading to depression, anxiety, and, in some cases, even suicidal thoughts.

At that moment, I knew we were facing a challenge that went beyond just treating his physical symptoms. We had to address the emotional and psychological aspects of his chronic pain.

Chronic pain is complex—it doesn't just stay in the body. For many patients like Mr. Turner, it infiltrates every part of life, altering their mood, their perception of themselves, and their relationships. Here's how we worked with Mr. Turner to help him manage his condition in a holistic way:

1. **Pain Management and Medication:** Turner had been prescribed a range of medications to help manage his chronic pain, including **opioids**, **NSAIDs**, and **muscle relaxants**. However, the key was to balance the medication carefully. Pain relief was necessary, but we also had to avoid dependency and side effects that could worsen his mood or cause other health problems. In collaboration with his GP and pain management team, we monitored his doses and made sure he was

also participating in non-pharmacological pain relief techniques, like physical therapy and gentle stretching exercises.

2. **Cognitive Behavioral Therapy (CBT) for Pain Management:** For many patients dealing with chronic pain, the brain and body become locked in a cycle of pain and negative thinking. **Cognitive Behavioral Therapy (CBT)** has proven highly effective for chronic pain sufferers because it helps break this cycle. We referred Turner to a **CBT therapist** who specialises in chronic pain management. Through CBT, Turner started to learn how his thoughts and emotions were amplifying his perception of pain. He began to recognize that while the pain wasn't going to disappear overnight, his emotional response to it could change. Slowly, he began to develop coping mechanisms, such as mindfulness and relaxation techniques, which helped him manage his pain better without feeling completely overwhelmed by it.

3. **Physical Therapy and Gentle Movement:** One of the greatest challenges for elderly patients with chronic pain is the fear of movement. Turner's pain made him hesitant to engage in any physical activity, fearing it would make the pain worse. However, **physical therapy** became a vital part of his treatment. We introduced Mr. Turner to a physiotherapist who worked with him to strengthen his muscles through gentle, targeted exercises. By gradually increasing his mobility, we aimed to reduce the physical strain on his joints and muscles. Over time, the physical therapist helped Mr. Turner rebuild his confidence in movement, showing him that some pain was not a signal to stop, but an indication to engage with his body in a more controlled way.

4. **Addressing Isolation and Depression:** Chronic pain often leads to isolation. Many patients feel ashamed

or embarrassed about needing help, leading them to withdraw from their family and friends. For Turner, the psychological impact of his chronic pain was just as crippling as the physical pain itself. We worked closely with the **psychology team** to address his growing depression. Turner had lost his desire to socialise or engage in activities he once enjoyed. Through **counselling**, we helped him reconnect with his interests and passions. We also encouraged his family to visit more often, providing both emotional support and practical assistance.

5. **Community Support and Social Services:** Many elderly people with chronic pain struggle to access community support or services, either due to mobility issues or the stigma of needing help. We connected Mr. Turner with local services that provided both social and practical support. His family were introduced to a **local carers' group**, where they could meet others in similar situations, share their experiences, and receive advice. Turner also joined a **community group for elderly men**, where he could talk about his experiences and build new friendships. It was essential that he felt part of the wider community and not isolated in his struggle.

Chronic pain is a condition that affects many older adults, but the psychological effects can often be ignored. For many elderly people, pain doesn't just affect their body—it affects their sense of self-worth, their relationships, and their outlook on life. For those who are struggling with chronic pain, it's important to remember that you don't have to face it alone. There is help available —through pain management, psychological support, physical rehabilitation, and community services.

Chronic pain is a major issue in the UK, particularly among the elderly. Fortunately, there are several resources available to help manage both the physical and psychological aspects of chronic pain:

- **NHS Pain Management Services:** The NHS offers a variety of pain management programs for those suffering from chronic pain. These include access to **specialist pain clinics**, where patients can receive multidisciplinary care, including medication management, physiotherapy, psychological therapy, and more.
- **Chronic Pain Support Groups:** Support groups for individuals living with chronic pain provide a space to share experiences and coping strategies. These can be local, in-person groups, or online forums, where people can connect with others in similar situations.
- **Cognitive Behavioral Therapy (CBT):** CBT has proven effective for helping individuals manage chronic pain by addressing the negative thoughts and behaviours associated with it. It's available through the NHS or privately through organisations like **Pain Concern**.
- **Carer's Support Groups:** Carers who look after those with chronic pain often face their own emotional and physical challenges. Support groups, like those run by **Carers UK**, provide a platform for carers to connect and share advice.
- **Physiotherapy and Occupational Therapy:** These services offer both practical and therapeutic support for managing chronic pain. Physiotherapists work to strengthen muscles and improve mobility, while occupational therapists can help people adjust their living environments to manage their pain more effectively.

❋ ❋ ❋

This chapter has explored the profound impact that chronic pain can have, not just on the body, but on the mind. For many elderly individuals like Mr. Turner, the experience of chronic pain can lead to depression, isolation, and a sense of hopelessness. But with the right combination of medical care, psychological support, and community involvement, it's possible to regain some sense of control and rebuild a more fulfilling life.

❋ ❋ ❋

In the next chapter, we'll explore the challenges faced by a patient dealing with **Spectrophobia - the fear of mirrors**, focusing on how spectrophobia can take over every aspect of a person's life and the interventions that can help regain control.

CHAPTER 9: REFLECTIONS OF THE SOUL

> "The face is the mirror of the soul. But for those who bear the scars of war, even the mirror reflects a different story—one of pain, fear, and the struggle to be seen for who they truly are, not what they appear to be."

It was a chilly autumn morning when I first met Mr. Thomas, a man in his early forties with a presence that seemed almost larger than life, despite the deep, painful vulnerability that sat behind his eyes. He was referred to our community mental health team due to his struggles with **spectrophobia**, a severe fear of seeing his own reflection. His case was unique—not just because of the intensity of his phobia, but because his fear was tied to something much deeper: the physical and emotional scars left by his time in the military.

Mr. Thomas had served in the army during a conflict in the Middle East, where he was severely injured in an explosion. His face, once a strong and familiar reflection of his identity, had been left disfigured. His nose was barely recognisable, his skin marred with deep, jagged scars that stretched across his cheek and forehead. The physical damage was overwhelming, but the emotional toll was even greater. For years, he refused to look at himself in a mirror, convinced that the face he saw was a mask of monstrosity.

His spectrophobia—his overwhelming fear of his own reflection—had become a daily torment.

Mr. Thomas' condition had led him to live a life of self-imposed isolation. He avoided social situations, refusing to leave his home except when absolutely necessary. When he did go out, it was under the cover of a large hat or sunglasses. His phobia was so extreme that even seeing his reflection in a shop window or a passing car's side mirror would trigger panic attacks, leaving him feeling overwhelmed with shame and dread.

One afternoon, we decided to conduct a **home visit** to understand his living situation better. The team and I arrived at his small flat in a quiet part of the city. His door was cracked open, and as we stepped inside, the air was thick with a sense of discomfort. Mr. Thomas was seated in the living room, his face partially hidden behind a large cap and scarf, his eyes darting nervously from the floor to the windows.

At one point during our conversation, I made a subtle suggestion that we try to look into a mirror together, to work through the fear gradually. As soon as the idea was introduced, he stood up abruptly, his hands trembling. "I can't. I can't do it," he muttered. The panic in his voice was palpable. The thought of confronting his disfigurement was so terrifying that it almost became a physical barrier between us. We were at an impasse.

At that moment, I realised that this wasn't just about confronting his own image. His trauma was so deeply intertwined with his fear that it couldn't be solved with a simple solution. We needed to approach his recovery with patience, understanding, and a focus on healing both mind and body.

Spectrophobia, especially in cases like Mr. Thomas', isn't just a fear of mirrors or reflections. It's often rooted in something much more profound—**trauma**. Mr. Thomas' disfigurement, a direct result of his military service, had become a symbol of the horrors he had endured. His face, scarred and marked by war, served as a constant reminder of the life he had lived, a life filled with violence, loss, and regret.

Here's how we worked with Mr. Thomas to help him start the long process of recovery:

1. **Trauma-Informed Care:** The first step was to acknowledge the deep **psychological trauma** that underpinned his fear of his reflection. Spectrophobia wasn't just about the physical appearance of his scars —it was about the emotional weight they carried. We connected Mr. Thomas with a **trauma specialist** who used a combination of **Cognitive Behavioral Therapy (CBT)** and **Exposure Therapy** to help him process his military experiences and begin to heal. Slowly, he began to open up about the horrors he had witnessed and the guilt he carried. Through this therapy, we helped him understand that his scars did not define him as a person, nor did they reflect his worth.

2. **Gradual Exposure to Mirrors:** As part of Mr. Thomas' treatment plan, we decided to incorporate **gradual exposure** to mirrors, but with extreme sensitivity to his comfort level. Instead of overwhelming him with his reflection right away, we started with small, manageable steps. For the first few sessions, we had Mr. Thomas sit across from a mirror that was covered by a light cloth, allowing him to catch glimpses of his reflection without feeling overwhelmed. Over time, the cloth was removed in stages, with Mr. Thomas becoming more comfortable with what he saw. His anxiety started to diminish as he realised that while his reflection was different, it didn't change who he was on the inside.

3. **Focusing on Identity Beyond Physical Appearance:** One of the key challenges with spectrophobia is the belief that one's external appearance is a direct reflection of internal worth. With Mr. Thomas, we worked to shift the focus from his external image to his inner self. He had a lifetime of experiences, values, and beliefs that

were much more important than his appearance. We encouraged him to reconnect with hobbies and interests that were important to him before the war. He started to take part in local veteran support groups, where he could speak openly with others who had similar experiences. These groups not only offered him the chance to share his feelings but also helped him regain his confidence in social settings.

4. **Support Systems and Peer Connections:** Mr. Thomas' military background had left him isolated. He found it difficult to connect with civilians who couldn't understand his trauma. We encouraged him to reach out to veterans' support groups and **peer support networks**, where he could bond with others who had gone through similar experiences. These peer groups provided a sense of camaraderie and understanding that had been missing in his life for years. Through these connections, Mr. Thomas began to see himself not just as a man scarred by war, but as a survivor with a story to tell.

5. **Counselling for War-Related Trauma:** Beyond the physical scars of his disfigurement, Mr. Thomas carried emotional scars that were harder to see. He had flashbacks, nightmares, and a deep sense of survivor guilt. We referred him to a **counsellor** specialising in **Post-Traumatic Stress Disorder (PTSD)**, who worked with him on **eye movement desensitisation and reprocessing (EMDR)** therapy. This method helped him process traumatic memories and reduce the emotional intensity associated with them. Slowly, he began to reframe his narrative, moving from a place of shame and pain to a place of acceptance and healing.

The journey of healing from **spectrophobia** isn't quick or easy, and for many, it's tied to deeper, often painful experiences. In Mr. Thomas' case, his fear of his own reflection was not just about his appearance—it was about the trauma he carried from war. His story is a powerful reminder that mental health challenges are often interconnected with physical, emotional, and social experiences. For anyone dealing with a similar issue, it's important to understand that there is help, and there is hope.

In the UK, those struggling with spectrophobia and trauma have access to a wide range of support services:

- **NHS Psychological Therapies (IAPT):** The **Improving Access to Psychological Therapies (IAPT)** program provides **CBT** and other therapeutic interventions for individuals struggling with anxiety, phobias, and trauma. Patients can be referred by their GP or self-refer online.
- **Veterans' Mental Health Services:** For military veterans like Mr. Thomas, the NHS offers specialised mental health services, such as the **Veterans' Mental Health Transition, Intervention and Liaison Service (TILS).** This service provides support for veterans dealing with trauma, PTSD, and other mental health conditions linked to their time in service.
- **War Trauma Support Groups:** There are numerous support groups and community organisations that cater to veterans. These groups offer peer support, counselling, and community activities that help veterans regain a sense of belonging and self-worth.
- **Private Therapy Providers:** In addition to NHS services, there are private therapists and counsellors who specialise in trauma and phobias. Many offer **EMDR** therapy, which has been shown to be effective in treating trauma and phobias.

※ ※ ※

In this chapter, we explored Mr. Thomas' journey through his battle with **spectrophobia**, a condition deeply rooted in both his physical disfigurement and his traumatic experiences as a soldier. While his fear of mirrors was overwhelming, his path to healing was a gradual one, guided by trauma-informed care, peer support, and therapy. This chapter serves as a reminder that healing is possible, even when the scars are both physical and emotional.

❊ ❊ ❊

In the next chapter, we will look at the case of **another patient**—a woman who faced overwhelming **guilt and isolation** after being diagnosed with a chronic illness, and how she found a way to reclaim her sense of self-worth.

CHAPTER 10: THE WEIGHT OF GUILT

> *"Sometimes, the hardest battle is not the physical pain, but the emotional struggle that comes with feeling broken."*

Chronic illness is a silent burden—one that often goes unnoticed by the outside world but weighs heavily on the individual. It's not just the physical symptoms that can consume a person; the emotional toll can be just as, if not more, overwhelming. Guilt, isolation, and a loss of self-worth can creep in and make each day feel like an insurmountable challenge.

This chapter focuses on the story of Sarah, a woman in her mid-thirties who was diagnosed with **rheumatoid arthritis**, a chronic condition that causes pain, swelling, and stiffness in the joints. When I met Sarah, she was living in the shadow of her diagnosis, grappling with the emotional consequences of her illness. It wasn't just the physical pain of her condition that kept her up at night—it was the guilt she felt for not being the person she once was, for feeling like a burden to her family, and for losing her sense of self-worth.

When Sarah was first referred to our community mental health team, she was reluctant to engage with anyone. She was a woman who had once thrived in her career, full of energy and ambition, but now she spent most of her time alone at home, feeling trapped in her body. Her chronic illness had rendered her physically weaker, and with each flare-up, her sense of independence seemed to slip further away. What struck me most during our first conversation was the **guilt** that hung over her like a dark cloud.

"I just feel like I'm letting everyone down," she said, her voice barely a whisper. "I can't do the things I used to do. I can't be the person I was before. I feel like a burden."

It was clear that Sarah's guilt wasn't just about the inconvenience of her condition; it was about how she saw herself in relation to the people around her. She felt as though she was failing in her role as a partner, a daughter, and a friend. The guilt of not being able to live life as she once had made her retreat further into isolation, afraid of being judged or pitied.

Sarah's condition had become an emotional prison. The chronic pain, while debilitating, was only part of the story. It was her internal struggle that held her captive.

Sarah's road to recovery began with understanding that her guilt, while natural, was misplaced. She wasn't a burden. She was not defined by her illness. The first step in her healing process was helping her **reframe her narrative**. Chronic illness often leads people to believe that they are no longer valuable or worthy of love and care. It's easy to lose sight of one's inherent worth when the world around you changes so drastically. But part of recovery lies in **reclaiming self-worth**—recognising that even in the face of chronic illness, there is still so much of you that remains intact.

1. **Challenging Negative Beliefs:** We started by exploring Sarah's **cognitive patterns**, specifically the belief that she was "less than" because of her illness. In Cognitive Behavioral Therapy (CBT), we work to uncover and challenge negative thoughts that contribute to feelings of guilt and inadequacy. Sarah's thought process had become distorted, as many people with chronic conditions experience. She believed that her illness made her weak and less valuable as a person. Through therapy, we began to break down those

thoughts, replacing them with healthier, more balanced perspectives.

2. **Building a Support Network:** One of the biggest challenges Sarah faced was her isolation. She stopped reaching out to friends and family because she didn't want to burden them with her problems. We worked on encouraging her to re-establish her support network, not only as a means of emotional support but as a reminder that she was still a valuable part of her community. Slowly, she began to open up about her fears and struggles with her loved ones, allowing them to offer the support she had been denying herself.

3. **Small Achievements, Big Wins:** For Sarah, even the smallest task became an overwhelming challenge due to her pain. We set small, achievable goals that could help her regain a sense of control and accomplishment. Whether it was cooking a meal for her family, going for a short walk, or simply getting dressed in the morning, we celebrated each victory, no matter how small it seemed. With each achievement, Sarah began to see herself as more than just her illness. She was still capable of contributing, of loving, and of living.

4. **Self-Compassion and Acceptance:** One of the hardest lessons for Sarah was learning **self-compassion**. She had been so hard on herself, expecting to be the same vibrant, active person she was before her diagnosis. But chronic illness doesn't fit neatly into any preconceived idea of how life should be. We worked on helping Sarah accept her condition without allowing it to define her entire sense of self. This acceptance didn't mean giving up hope or resigning to her illness—it meant recognizing her limitations while also acknowledging her strengths and resilience.

5. **Engaging in Meaningful Activities:** Lastly, we encouraged Sarah to return to some of the activities that once brought her joy, but in a modified form. For

Sarah, this meant finding new hobbies that she could do at home, like painting and creative writing. Engaging in creative activities helped her tap into a source of joy that wasn't tied to her physical abilities. As Sarah began to reclaim her sense of purpose, her guilt diminished, and her emotional well-being improved.

For individuals like Sarah who are grappling with chronic illness and the emotional toll it takes, there are various support systems and resources available:

- **NHS Mental Health Services:** Chronic illness often requires a multidisciplinary approach, including both medical and mental health support. The NHS offers **Cognitive Behavioral Therapy (CBT)** for individuals dealing with **chronic illness**, anxiety, and depression. CBT can help reframe negative thoughts and improve coping mechanisms.
- **Chronic Illness Support Groups:** There are numerous online and in-person support groups for people living with chronic conditions such as arthritis, fibromyalgia, and other long-term illnesses. These groups provide a sense of community, allowing individuals to share their experiences and offer support to one another.
- **Pain Management Clinics:** For those struggling with the physical pain of chronic illness, **pain management clinics** across the UK provide expert care in helping to manage symptoms and improve quality of life. These clinics often offer physical therapies, medication management, and psychological support.
- **Mindfulness and Stress Reduction Programs:** Mindfulness-based stress reduction (MBSR) programs can help individuals living with chronic illness manage stress, reduce anxiety, and cultivate self-compassion. These programs are available through various providers in the UK and can be beneficial for managing both physical and emotional symptoms.
- **Macmillan Cancer Support:** For individuals with chronic

illness related to cancer or cancer treatment, **Macmillan** offers a wide range of services, from counselling and emotional support to practical help with managing daily challenges.

❋ ❋ ❋

Sarah's journey is a powerful reminder that while chronic illness may change the way we live, it doesn't diminish our value as individuals. Through therapy, self-compassion, and rebuilding her support network, Sarah was able to reclaim her self-worth and find new ways to enjoy life despite her condition.

ACKNOWLEDGMENTS

This book is the culmination of many stories shared by patients, colleagues, and friends who have all contributed to my understanding of mental health in profound ways. Each individual's journey has taught me something invaluable about resilience, healing, and the human spirit.

I would like to thank my colleagues and mentors in the mental health field for their continued support, guidance, and wisdom. I am also deeply grateful to the patients I've had the privilege to work with; their courage and vulnerability have inspired me more than words can express.

Lastly, I want to thank my family and partner for their unwavering love and encouragement throughout the process of writing this book. Their belief in me and the work I do has been a constant source of strength.

This book is for anyone who has ever struggled, felt invisible, or thought that they were alone in their journey.

❋ ❋ ❋

YOU ARE NOT.

ABOUT THE AUTHOR

Mcarthur Okorocha

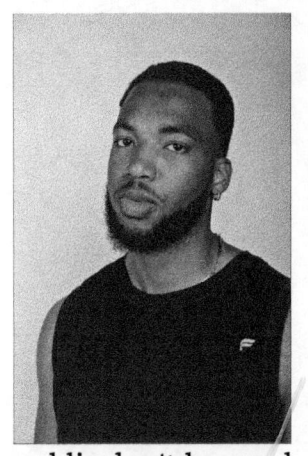 McArthur Okorocha is a mental health nursing student with a career in mental health spanning over 4 years. During the pandemic in 2020 he discovered a drive to self-improve and learn more about mental health after going through a loss of job and suffering from depression himself.

This book was inspired by his experiences from working in the mental health community and noticing how much the public don't know about different disorders, whilst also shedding light on stigmas that needs to be corrected. McArthur lives in London and can be found on Instagram and Tiktok at @4uche. If you'd like to get in touch, please contact macthebusiness@gmail.com

www.ingramcontent.com/pod-product-compliance
Lightning Source LLC
Chambersburg PA
CBHW070418230526
45471CB00006B/2869